Menopause Sympto

Menopause gei
woman's late 40s   .y 50s,
however, the avera   . age is
approximately 51. You are officially in
menopause after you have gone without
a menstrual period for at least one year.
In the years leading up to menopause,
you are said to be in peri-menopause,
and it is during this time that you many
start experiencing bothersome
menopausal symptoms, due to
fluctuating levels of circulating hormone
levels.

Common Menopause Symptoms

The symptoms and severity of peri-
menopause and menopause vary
among individuals, however, a great

majority of women experience hot flashes, night sweats, vaginal dryness, mood swings and irregular menstrual bleeding. The bleeding may be scant, or very heavy. In fact, a condition known as dysfunctional uterine bleeding (DUB) is very common in the years leading to menopause, and can be so severe, that it sometimes leads to anemia. In these cases, oral iron supplements are often effective in normalizing iron stores. In addition, genetics and family history may play an important role in the type and severity of menopause symptoms that you experience. Furthermore, the age at which you reach menopause may also be reflective of the age your mother was when she entered menopause.

Surgical vs. Natural Menopause

If you go through natural menopause, your menopause symptoms will typically be milder, than if you go through a surgically or chemically induced menopause. Surgical menopause happens when the ovaries are removed during a hysterectomy. If only the uterus is removed, but the ovaries retained, premature menopause is less likely to occur. Chemical menopause occurs as a result of certain cancer treatments. The abruptness of surgical and chemical menopause often cause profound hot flashes and night sweats, which can be very disruptive to your life. Fortunately, regardless of whether you are going through natural menopause, surgical or chemical menopause, there are a number of highly effective treatment options that can help relieve your symptoms.

Hot Flashes and Night Sweats

Two of the most common menopause symptoms are hot flashes or flushes, and night sweats. Hot flashes causes intense feelings of heat, sometimes accompanied by facial flushing and redness. These menopause symptoms are caused by a vasomotor response, and can last anywhere from 1 to 10 years. In fact, some women experience vasomotor symptoms until well into there 70s, and some women are affected their entire lives, albeit with less frequency and intensity. They are also commonly accompanied by profuse sweating of the head and neck areas, palpitations and dizziness. Some women are so negatively influenced by hot flashes, that they experience panic attacks. When hot flashes occur at night, they are known as night sweats. Night sweats disrupt your sleep and you might also find yourself getting up to change your pajamas because they are drenched with sweat.

Hormone Replacement Therapy

Hormone replacement therapy, or HRT effectively relieves hot flashes and night sweats, but they are not appropriate for everyone. Those with a personal or family history of gynecological cancers such as breast, uterine, ovarian or endometrial cancer should not take hormones. Many gynecological cancers are fueled by estrogen, and when you take replacement hormones to relieve your menopause symptoms, cancerous cells may be spurred into growth. Hormone replace therapy may also be inappropriate for those with a personal or family history of cardiovascular disease, blood clots, stroke or high blood pressure. Also, if you smoke, you may not be a candidate for hormone replacement therapy because the combination may raise your risk for a stroke. Home remedies that may help relieve hot flashes and night sweats include avoiding caffeine and spicy foods, not smoking, maintaining your weight, wearing breathable fabric clothing and keeping your bedroom cool. Also, stress management techniques such as meditation, deep breathing, yoga and aromatherapy may prove beneficial as well.

Phytoestrogens

Flaxseed and soybeans contain rich amounts of phytoestrogens, which are naturally occurring estrogen-like substances that mimic the effects of your body's natural estrogen stores. Other foods that contain phytoestrogens include peanuts, wheat, cashews, corn and apples. Consuming these foods may ease your menopause symptoms of hot flashes, night sweats and vaginal dryness. Phytoestrogens are excellent sources of isoflavanoids, which are similar in chemical composition to natural estrogen. Not only do phytoestrogens help fight damage caused by free radicals, they also help block or inhibit the effects of too much circulating estrogen. When you have excess circulating estrogen in your body, you may be at a higher risk for developing certain gynecological cancers such as those of the breast and uterus. Although considered safe when consumed in moderation, eating a diet high in phytoestrogens may also promote benign cystic changes in the breast and reproductive organs. Talk to your doctor before including soy or other phytoestrogen products into your diet, or before you consider taking soy supplements.

Omega-3 Fatty Acids

Omega-3 fatty acids, found in fresh, fatty fish such as salmon, tuna and mackerel, have shown promise in the treatment of hot flashes and night sweats. Not only do omega-3 fatty acids help reduce the intensity and frequency of hot flashes and night sweats, they may also be beneficial in the management of menopausal-related depression, anxiety, insomnia and mood swings. Since these fish oils have potent anticoagulant properties, they may intensify the effects of aspirin or prescription anticoagulant medications. Although getting omega-3 fatty acids through diet is considered safe, consuming them via supplementation may cause unusual or abnormal bleeding Before taking fish oil or omega-

3 fatty acid supplements, talk to your doctor to make sure they are appropriate for your situation. It is important to note, that although effective, you may not notice immediate benefits from fish oil because it often takes approximately three weeks for results to be noticed.

Antidepressants

Antidepressants are sometimes prescribed to manage hot flashes and night sweats for those who are unable, or who prefer not to take hormone replacement therapy. They are also effective in treating menopausal-related depression, and may also improve your quality of sleep. Although antidepressants are not known to increase the risk of certain gynecological cancers in the way that hormone replacement therapy may, they can cause significant side effects. Side effects from antidepressants may include palpitations, weight gain, insomnia, anxiety, dizziness and headache.

Restoring Vaginal Moisture

Vaginal dryness and atrophy are also common menopause symptoms. As levels of estrogen decline, the vaginal mucosa loses elasticity and moisture which leads to irritation, itching, dryness, and sometimes bleeding. Staying well-hydrated by drinking plenty of water helps tissues stay moist, however, this is often not enough.

Hormonal preparations that are inserted vaginally work well to restore moisture and atrophied tissue, and unlike oral hormone replacement therapy, there is less of a risk of adverse reaction and long-term health consequences.

Transdermal or vaginal testosterone cream may also help restore the vaginal tissue without creating levels of elevated systemic estrogen. Over-the-counter personal lubricants also help relieve symptoms, and some are even formulated to promote optimal vaginal flora, while helping to repair atrophied tissue. Botanicals such as black cohosh may help thicken the vaginal mucosa so that it is not as prone to dryness, fissures, cracks and bleeding. Dandelion leaves, a common herb may also help restore moisture and lubrication to the vaginal tissue. As with any other menopause treatment, seek the advice of your health care provider before self-treating with botanicals or herbal remedies.

Osteoporosis

The risk of osteoporosis also rises as women reach menopause. Estrogen helps keep bones strong, and when estrogen levels decline, women become more at risk for developing brittle bones and fractures. Calcium and vitamin D supplements may help support bone health, but taking too much can cause a dangerous condition known as hypercalcemia, or high levels of calcium in the blood. Over time, high levels of blood calcium may raise the risk for the development of calcium deposits in the blood vessels, increasing the risk for cardiovascular disease. Getting your calcium from food sources do not seem to carry the same risks as supplements, so talk to your doctor about which sources of calcium and vitamin D he recommends. Vitamin C helps with collagen repair and synthesis. Although many medical professionals recommend 2,000 mg of vitamin C per day, this dosage may cause stomach upset, heartburn and diarrhea. It may be better tolerated when taken in divided doses.

Dry Skin and Eyes

Dry eyes and dry skin may also develop during the menopausal years. The eyes often feel itchy and gritty, and the sensation is generally worse in the morning. Dry, itchy skin may also worsen during menopause, and is also the result of declining estrogen levels. Stay well-hydrated by drinking plenty of water helps restore moisture to the mucus membranes and skin. Using moistening eye drops is also helpful in treating dry eyes, and taking lukewarm oatmeal baths helps skin retain moisture. Moisturizing your skin with a rich lotion relieves dryness and itching, and is more effective when applied soon after a bath or shower. Do not take excessively hot baths or showers because this further dries out your skin. Also, limiting your intake of caffeinated beverages may also help keep your skin from becoming too dry. Certain dietary supplements such as fish oil and flaxseed also help keep skin soft and supple. These supplements may also help reduce the risk of breast cancer, however, before taking them talk to your doctor.

Urinary Problems

Loss of estrogen can also contribute to bladder prolapse, urinary leaking and urinary frequency. Urinary incontinence, which is another common complaint of menopausal women, is one of the more embarrassing symptoms of menopause. Hormone replacement therapy helps restore estrogen stores and can dramatically reduce the incidence of leaking, frequency and incontinence. Urinary tract infections may also become more freqeunt during menopause, so drinking plenty of water to maintain bladder health, and drinking cranberry juice may help keep the urinary tract less vulnerable to bacterial infections. When hormone replacement therapy is not an option, there are other natural treatments than can help. Keeping your weight within normal limits and avoiding caffeine may help stop bladder problems, as might doing pelvic floor exercises known as Kegal exercises. To learn how to do Kegal exercises, pretend that you are voiding, and in mid-stream, try to stop the flow of urine. Contracting and releasing these muscles helps make them stronger so that urinary leaking will be less likely.

Mood Swings

If you experience frequent mood swings, you're not alone. Research has shown that omega-3 fatty acids can significantly help brighten your mood, while helping to release your body's "feel good" chemicals known as endorphins. Vitamin D, which is actually a hormone, can also help increase the production of certain chemicals in the brain known to improve mood. Of course, getting enough exercise and staying socially connect also helps keep bad moods in check. When your mood does not improve, despite natural remedies, a course of antidepressants may help get you back on track. Not only will antidepressants help improve your mood, they may also help relieve hot flashes and night sweats. Mood swings can also contribute to anxiety and panic attacks. Taking a low-dose magnesium supplement may help keep you calm and anxiety-free. Magnesium citrate is better absorbed than magnesium oxide, however, it may cause loose stools. Magnesium also helps enhance a better quality of sleep, and has also shown to decrease hot flashes and night sweats. It also helps relieve muscle aches and pains that sometimes occur during menopause, and might even help stave off depression. Talk to your doctor before taking magnesium supplements because they may interfere with certain medications that you're taking, or they might be contraindicated with certain medical conditions.

Palpitations

Many menopausal women complain about heart palpitations. These can be especially alarming when they begin, out of nowhere. They sometimes occur after eating, but often occur in conjunction with hot flashes. They are generally nothing to be concerned about, however, they can indicate problems with the cardiovascular system. Heart disease generally rises with age, and is more pronounced in the post-menopausal years. Women who have had their ovaries removed during hysterectomy may be at a higher risk for heart disease than women who still have their ovaries. The ovaries are the body's main source of estrogen, and estrogen may be cardioprotective. To reduce the intensity and frequency of palpitations, consider taking magnesium citrate supplements. Known as "nature's beta blocker," magnesium helps regulate the heart rate and it also helps keep blood pressure within normal limits. Eating smaller, more frequent meals can also help stave off palpitations that occur after meals. Avoiding caffeine, smoking, managing stress and getting regular exercise also helps relieve palpitations. Certain medications can contribute to palpitations as well. These include decongestants, antidepressants, certain pain medications and some antihistamines. Although common during menopause, if palpitations are accompanied by shortness of breath, chest pain, dizziness, swollen ankles or numbness, seek emergency medical treatment. When natural treatments for palpitations fail to bring relief, medications such as propranolol can help slow the heart rate to eliminate palpitations. Propranolol does have side effects, however. They include fatigue, dizziness, exercise intolerance, insomnia, slow pulse, nasal congestion, constipation and cold extremities. Most of these side effects are temporary, however, and tend to dissipate after a few weeks. In addition, most side effects from propranolol are dose dependent, so if your do experience side effects, your doctor can decrease your dosage, which will help eliminate them. Making sure that you get enough potassium in your diet is also good for your heart, and may help regulate your heart's rate and rhythm. Eating foods rich in potassium such as bananas and oranges helps keep palpitations as bay, and it also helps maintain a normal blood pressure.

Tingling And Electric Shock Sensations

One of the more stranger symptoms linked to menopause is a tingling or electric shock sensation that is felt in the extremities. Although the hands and feet are most often affected, numbness and tingling can occur anywhere in the body, including the face, head, mouth, vaginal area, the breasts and even the eyes. These symptoms are usually the result of lowered levels of circulating estrogen, and women often report that these tingling sensations feel like prickly, creeping feelings. This sensation is known as formication, and although commonly associated with menopause, formication can also be caused by vitamin deficiencies, diabetes, potassium or calcium deficiencies, anxiety and problems with circulations. To rule any medical conditions, see your doctor if you experience numbness or tingling in your extremities, or any other parts of your body. Stabilizing your hormones with hormone replacement therapy often relieves tingling, however again, it is not appropriate for certain women. Eating a healthy diet and exercising daily can improve formication because when your body is healthy, you are less likely to experience the effects of hormonal fluctuations. Because magnesium helps calm nerve fibers and muscles, taking a magnesium citrate supplement may help with tingling, especially if your symptoms are associated with stress.

Changes In Hair Growth

Of course, women love a luxurious head of healthy hair, but nobody wants an increase in facial hair. Unfortunately, this sometimes happens as a result of menopause. Your changing hormone levels can also cause you to experience thinning hair on your scalp, legs and underarms. Certain medications commonly taking during the menopausal years can also contribute to hair loss, and they include, but are not limited to , beta blockers and certain hormonal preparations. Using a mild shampoo, and avoiding hairstyles that cause tension on the hair can help avoid hair fallout. If hair loss becomes overly noticeable, products such as Rogaine can help spur hair growth. Talk to your doctor before using this product because it may interact negatively with certain medications, or cause side effects. Hypothyroidism, which is also common during menopause can also cause hair loss, however, other symptoms are often noticed first. These include weight gain or the inability to lose weight, hoarseness, dry skin, puffy eyelids, constipation, feeling cold, fatigue, elevated blood lipid levels, heavy menstrual periods and a slow pulse. Treating hypothyroidism with thyroid replacement therapy often brings rapid relief to symptoms.

Muscle And Joint Pain

Muscle and joint pain is another frequent complaint of menopausal women. Pains in the neck, shoulders, back, hips, knees, ankles and feet are common, as are headaches, jaw pain and rib pain. Eating foods rich in calcium and vitamin D are often helpful in relieve muscle and joint discomfort, as is engaging in regular exercise. Taking Epsom salt baths is very soothing, and often brings substantial relief from those affected by menopause-related musculoskeletal manifestations. Epsom salts are rich in magnesium, which helps improve nerve and muscle function, while relaxing tense muscles. The etiology behind menopausal-related muscle and joint pain remains unclear, however, it is thought that reduced levels of estrogen plays an important role in the development of these symptoms. Estrogen affects muscles and joints by keeping inflammation to a minimum, so therefore, as levels of estrogen decline in the years leading up to menopause, the joints get less amounts of estrogen, resulting in pain and inflammation. For certain women, the joint pain and stiffness is worse in the morning, while swelling is worse as the day wears on. Menopausal weight gain can also exacerbate aches and pains, not only because excess weight exerts pressure on the joints, but because being overweight may trigger an inflammatory response as well. Although exercise is often recommended to ease discomfort, some women are unable to tolerate its effects. Certain women who are prone to menopausal muscle aches and joint pain might experience intense, shooting pains down the arms or legs, especially after an exercise session. If this occurs, it is important to speak to your health care provider to rule out other causes for your pain. Exercise is very important, especially during menopause, so that exercise becomes more tolerable. Non-steroidal anti-inflammatory drugs (NSAIDs) are particularly useful in mitigating joint pain. These medications include ibuprofen, naproxen sodium and aspirin. If you are unable to tolerate side effects such as stomach upset, or if you are taking prescription anticoagulant medications, taking NSAIDs may not be an appropriate treatment option for you. Acetaminophen, the active ingredient in Tylenol can also help relieve pain, however, unlike NSAIDs, acetaminophen does little to reduce inflammation. Gentle massage is also highly effective in relieving muscle soreness and joint pain. It not only promotes muscle relaxation, it also promotes optimal circulation, which helps in the healing process.

To further relieve pain and stiffness related to menopause, visit your health care provider first, to determine the exact cause of your pain. Staying active and fit helps keep your joints strong and flexible, so consider incorporating yoga or tai chi into your routine exercise regimen. Of course, decreasing pressure on your weight bearing joints such as your hips and knees by keeping your weight within normal limits also helps, as does trying to avoid repetitive strain on your joints.

Managing your stress levels is also very important in the treatment of muscle and joint pain. When you are under stress, your body releases a hormone known as cortisol, which can contribute to inflammation. Prolonged stress may cause inflammation to rapidly spread, worsening your pain. Lifestyle modifications such as regular exercise may help regulate your levels of cortisol to reduce inflammation. In addition, limiting your intake of sugar and carbohydrates can also keep you more comfortable. Chronic inflammation and subsequent pain can be caused by consuming a diet high in sugar, white bread, flour and rice. Also, a high carbohydrate diet can also promote insulin irregularities, which can disrupt cellular metabolism and worsen inflammation. Eating certain fruits such as cherries, blackberries and blueberries can have a dramatic effect on your level of pain. These fruits are rich sources of antioxidants and anti-inflammatories which are very beneficial in the management of inflammation and pain.

Gum Problems

Gum problems such as gingivitis are also common menopause symptoms. Again, the fluctuations in hormones is thought to be responsible for gum disease during menopause. Swollen, red and bleeding gums are common, so brushing and flossing at least twice a day is important in maintaining oral health. If gingivitis is not managed effectively, it can progress into a condition known as periodontitis, which may cause destruction of the bones that hold your teeth in place, and result in tooth loss. Eating a diet rich in fruits, vegetables, fiber and lean proteins help maintain oral health, as does drinking plenty of water to rinse away bacteria, avoiding junk food and not smoking. If you have gingivitis, you gums may bleed more when you floss.

They may even bleed spontaneously, however, do not let this deter you from flossing every time you brush. Flossing, despite the bleeding, will strengthen your gums, and help remove bacteria-causing plaque from your teeth and gum line. Taking a vitamin C supplement may also promote oral health, however, before you take supplements, talk to your dental professional.

Take Away Message

Everyone experiences menopause differently. While some women face symptomatic challenges, others sail through it with hardly a hot flash. Maintaining a healthy lifestyle and keeping an open dialogue with your health care provider can help you manage your menopause symptoms in the best way possible.

12601601R00022

Printed in Great Britain
by Amazon.co.uk, Ltd.,
Marston Gate.